Brenda's Bible

ALSO BY BRENDA KINSEL

40 over 40:
40 Things Every Woman Over 40 Needs
to Know About Getting Dressed

In the Dressing Room with Brenda:
A Fun and Practical Guide to Buying
Smart and Looking Great

Brenda's Wardrobe Companion:
A Guide to Getting Dressed
from the Inside Out

Brenda's Bible

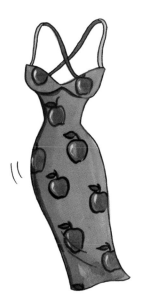

Escape Fashion Hell and Experience Heaven

Every Time You Get Dressed

BRENDA KINSEL

WILDCAT CANYON PRESS
An Imprint of Council Oak Books
San Francisco/Tulsa

Brenda's Bible
Escape Fashion Hell and Experience Heaven Every Time You Get Dressed

Brenda Kinsel

Illustration by Shannon Laskey

WILDCAT
CANYON
PRESS

Wildcat Canyon Press
An Imprint of Council Oak Books
San Francisco/Tulsa

Typographic specifications:
Body text set in Cochin, additional text set in Univers, and Handwriting

ISBN 1-885171-81-1

To my church buddy, Kim Kuhn, from your lucky
(and forever grateful) duckling

contents

acknowledgments

The idea for *Brenda's Bible* was conceived in a magical meeting involving Paulette Millichap, my publisher; Erin Kinsel, my 23-year-old daughter; Toni Bernbaum, my assistant; and myself. *Brenda's Wardrobe Companion* had just been published and we were tossing around ideas about how to support it in its early months, but Erin had been uncharacteristically quiet. Finally, Paulette said, "Erin, what do you think?" And out of the blue, Erin said, "I think it would be great to have a small book that people could carry in their handbags, take shopping with them, that would clearly lay out Brenda's rules for getting it right — you know, like a bible. Brenda's Bible."

Now, I want to thank the source of the magic — whatever it might be called — that was in the room that day, and also Council Oak's associate publisher, Ja-lene Clark, for actually putting a schedule to the project, keeping us all on it, and for her insights and hunches that always make for a better book. I thank Toni for her glee and her talent in knowing where to dig for the good stuff and how to knit it all together. Thanks also to the editing talent and manuscript organization of Tamara Traeder.

Big thanks to Jenny Phillips for the book cover, and to Shannon Laskey, whose illustrations made it all come alive and carry this book to Paradise.

My love and deep appreciation to my clients who continually inspire and delight me season after season. Working with you takes me right to heaven. To friends and family who jump in with support at all the right times, particularly the Bellas, my 7 @ 7 Group, the M & M's, and Mom and Dad.

And to Russ Gelardi, my sweetheart, for always taking time to give an expert's eye to copy and layout, offering great suggestions, but more importantly, for always being there for me, in love and in light.

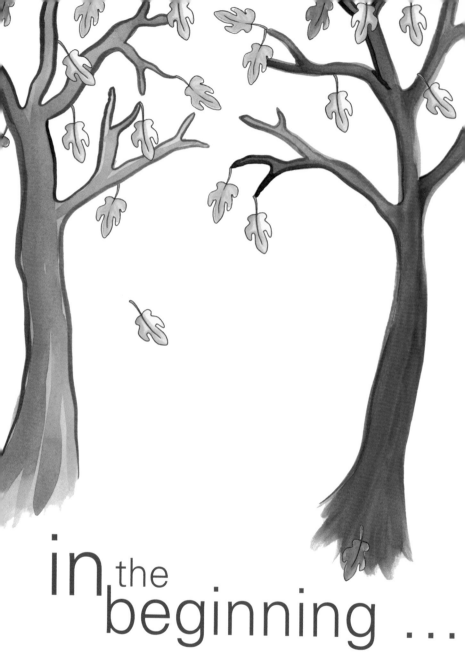

in the
beginning ...

. . . there were fig leaves — in small, medium, and large. Fig leaves for casual wear. Fig leaves for formal wear. It was simple. Today the choices are endless. We have constructed, un-constructed, and de-constructed clothing to choose from on department store racks. Stuffed inside our closets are items made from viscose, rayon, silk, wool, virgin wool, hemp, stretch linen, pleather, tulle, fancy polyester, and spandex. We mix floral prints with vintage plaids, pink leather with lace. And sometimes it works.

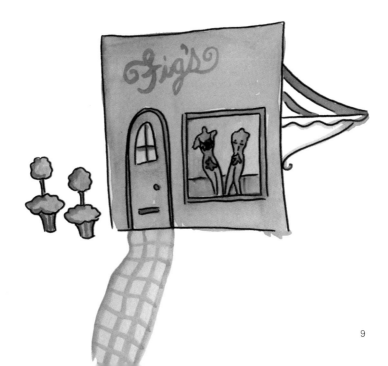

Back there, in the beginning, it was easy. Adam and Eve just lollygagged around Paradise all day with no one to impress, no parties to go to, no job interviews, no needing to get dressed to attract the opposite sex, no closet to organize. But no sooner were they booted out of the garden of Eden than they had to face the daily decision of what to wear with what and when to wear it. How do you go from work to meeting your in-laws without changing clothes? What do you wear to see the tax man? Is a flowing goddess dress too "over the top" for a birthday bash? Details, details, details! Receive a party invitation these days with a suggested dress code like "elegantly casual" or "creative black tie" and you want to slam your closet door, stay home, overdo it on the leftover apple crisp and pull the sheets up over your head. I don't blame you. It's a jungle in there — and I'm just talking about your closet. Pantyhose are tangled like snakes on the floor. Party clothes have collected an inch of dust on their shoulders. Plastic dry-cleaning bags are threatening to take over and strangle the good stuff. And no matter how full that closet is, have you noticed, you still have nothing to wear? You know where you are? You're in fashion hell.

The problems started out small. They always do. But now the red flames of despair are licking at your precious feet. You left for work knowing full well that the hem on your skirt was falling out, but you thought, "Oh, if I can just make it to the office, I'll get double-sided tape from the supply closet and tape it up!" But guess what — when you got there, there wasn't any! Your best client arrived, perfectly coiffed, and you felt crummy all day.

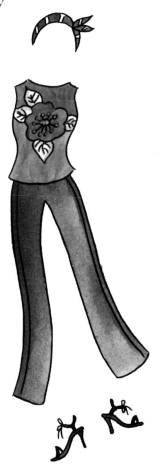

Or, maybe you say it's "shyness" that makes you turn down every social invitation, but secretly you only know how to dress for work and washing the car on the weekend. You have no idea how to dress for "fun" events, and you don't want to show up in something inappropriate and blow your cover.

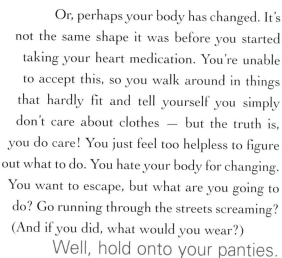

Or, perhaps your body has changed. It's not the same shape it was before you started taking your heart medication. You're unable to accept this, so you walk around in things that hardly fit and tell yourself you simply don't care about clothes — but the truth is, you do care! You just feel too helpless to figure out what to do. You hate your body for changing. You want to escape, but what are you going to do? Go running through the streets screaming? (And if you did, what would you wear?)

Well, hold onto your panties. There is a way out of this fiery pit. Fashion Heaven is close at hand, and so take my hand. I'll lead you through the valley of all those clothes that tempted you because they were on sale, all those outfits that make you feel drab or fat or like your mother (no offense, Mom). I'll get you through the fires of your worn-out look: and douse the flames of all those items that never quite fit. Come with me where you'll find green (in the shade that looks best on you) pastures where peace and confidence prevail, where problems with clothes disappear, and where you feel radiant getting dressed every day.

You think I'm fibbing? I'm not! I've helped redeem good women just like you who ended up in fashion hell.

They wrote me postcards and
called out for help.
See if any of their problems
ring a bell for you.

postcards
from
hell

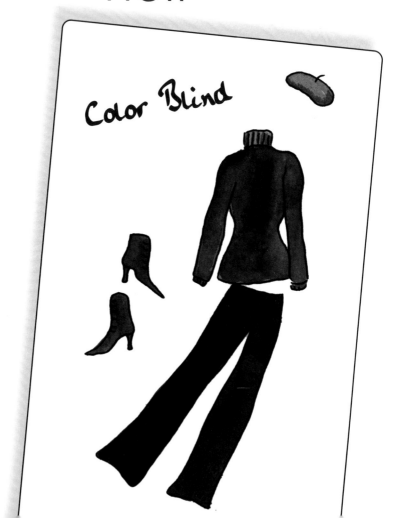

Color Blind

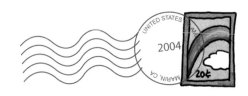

Dear Brenda,

I'm finally sick of black, but that's all I own. I'm living in a black and white world but my soul is screaming for rainbows in Technicolor.
I don't have a clue how to bring color into my life. When I go shopping, you know what I buy? Black. Over and over again. I know I've got to stop, but I can't.

Signed,
Color Blind

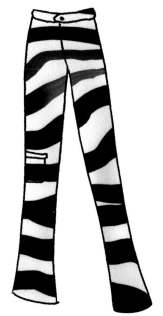

Hanging On By a Limb

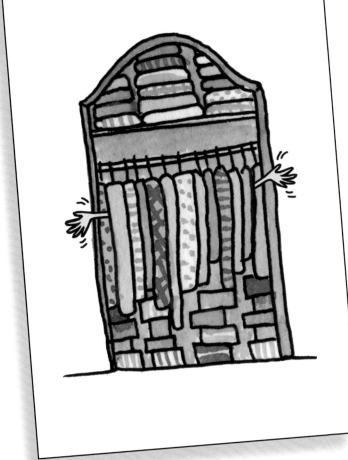

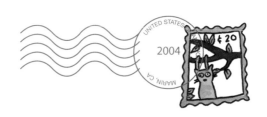

Dear Brenda,

My closet is a dangerous place. When I put my arm inside to pull something out, I have to wrestle with my clothes to get it back. Everything is packed in there so tight that even if I get a garment out, the wrinkles in it look permanent. It's hopeless. It's just easier to wear the same thing every day. A navy blue blazer, navy pants and a T-shirt. How boring. What's wrong with me?

Signed,
Hanging on By a Limb

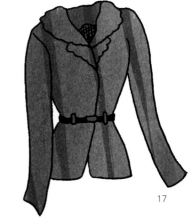

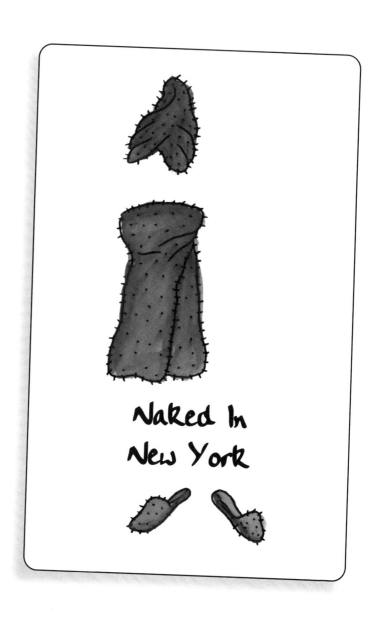

Naked In
New York

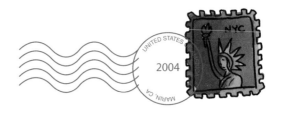

Dear Brenda ,

When I got to the hotel and pulled out the evening gown I was wearing to the awards ceremony, I discovered the sensor was still attached. Then I realized I forgot to shop for the thong underwear I needed to wear under the slinky fabric. These fashion details are ruining my life! Will I ever be a grownup and get it right?

Signed,
Naked in
New York

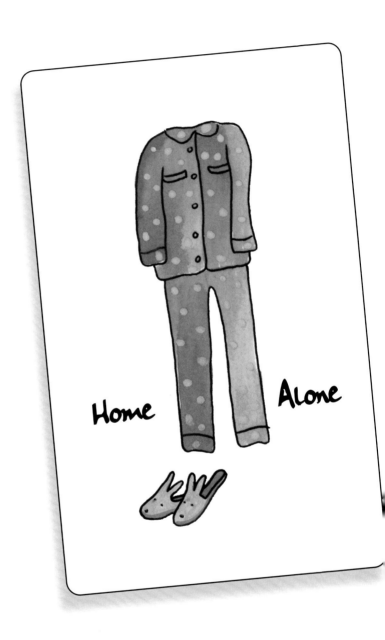

Home Alone

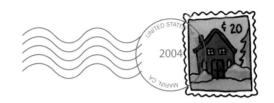

UNITED STATES

2004

MARIN, CA

$ 20

Dear Brenda,

I had the chance to meet my favorite actor at the opening of the local film festival tonight. Instead, I'm sitting here writing you this postcard. I don't know how to put anything together. I haven't kept up with my wardrobe, and now when I need it the most, it's failed me. No party clothes, nothing festive.
No action.

Signed,
Home Alone

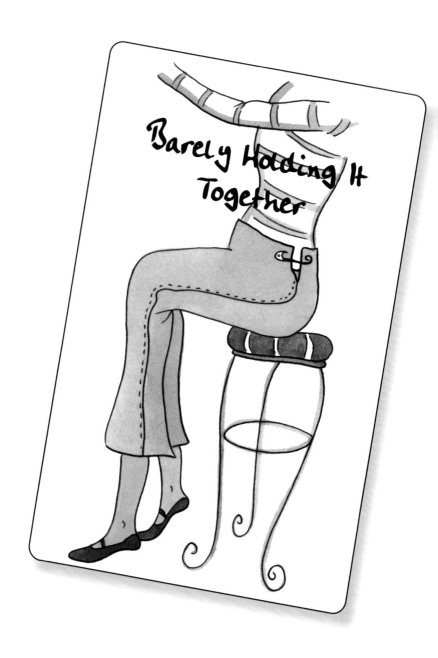

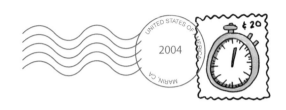

Dear Brenda,

I've outgrown all my clothes but I hate to shop so I'm holding my pants together with rubber bands, safety pins, and duct tape. My body is nothing like the bodies in magazines. I'll never look good in fashionable clothes. Why should I even try?

Signed,
Barely Holding
It Together

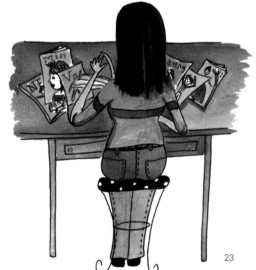

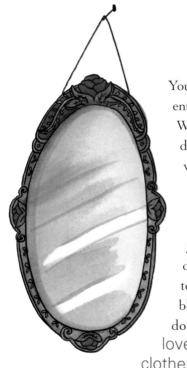

Your particular fashion hell might look different from the ones these women describe. Whether we experience despair in the dressing room or disgust in our closets, whether we grossly neglect our clothing needs or pretend that none of it really matters, we all have our own demons to wrestle with. Maybe you've numbed yourself to the problems of getting dressed with some talk about how you're too old, too fat, or too _____(fill in the blank) to care about clothes anyway. I don't believe you. Everyone would love the chance to look good in clothes, feel good in clothes, and wear clothes with confidence. Well, I'm here to tell you all that IS possible ... for you!

But let's get prepared for change. Sometimes it gets worse before it gets better. When you recognize the Seven Deadliest Fashion Sins, you'll probably discover maladies you didn't realize you had. But hey, chin up. I'm not going to take you someplace scary without a light to lead you out. And light the way I will with the Ten Fashion Commandments. You'll probably be so happy with these new guidelines that you'll want to testify, "I've been saved!"

You'll get a chance to come into the Fashion Confessional with me where you'll hear other people's predicaments followed by solutions that just might be the ones you've been praying for.

You'll see how to move gracefully through the fashion seasons. I'll show you how to create miracle makeovers in minutes or hours, depending on how much time you have. I'll reveal it all — the last word on shopping, fashion, and getting dressed. You're already on your way to discovering fashion heaven right here on earth. So read on, you'll be having so much fun in clothes, you might even think it's a sin. Be Daring. Trust me.

Let this book be the answer to your prayers.

the seven deadliest
fashion sins

The first thing I want to introduce you to is a list of the Seven Deadliest Fashion Sins. Just one of these Seven Deadlies has the power to kill any creativity or joy that comes with the act of getting dressed, when in fact, getting dressed should be the first (or at least nearly the first) creative and joyful thing you do each day.

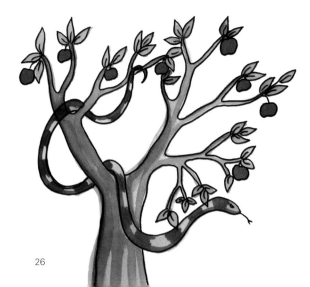

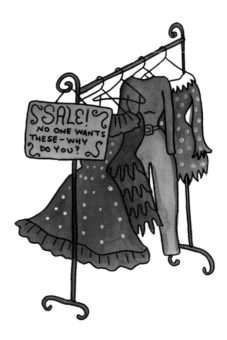

1. Delusion

If you buy what you can't fix — like the jacket that's sized for an NBA basketball player when you're the size of a ballet instructor, or the cute magenta blouse whose color would look great on you if you just bought all new makeup and dyed your hair — you're in a state of delusion. In spite of overwhelming evidence that it doesn't work, you continue to buy all those sale items that you think you'll wear (but never do). Your closet is not meant to be a shelter for sale items that no one else will take home. Falling for clothes that need major overhauls is as deadly as falling for the man who just needs a job and a sense of humor in order to be the right fit for you. Take off the blinders and get real. Train yourself to know what's really right for you right now.

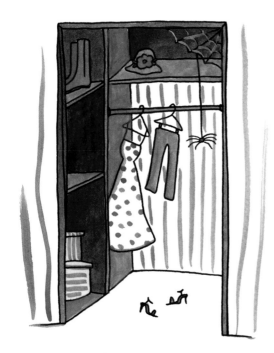

2. Neglect

Neglecting yourself and denying that clothes matter — "Oh, I don't care about clothes" — is the cover-up (and hardly stylish) for not taking the time to figure out how to please yourself with clothes. Unless you're either a nun and your habit is all laid out for you or you live in a nudist colony, your life requires clothes — so make it your mission to find the ones you love.

3. Idolatry

Many a woman is paralyzed by the defeat that comes with idolizing what she can't have. While she worships half her size, she can't enjoy her whole essence. While she covets expensive designer clothes, she can't let herself feel great in fashions she can afford. Size is only a number, not a measure of your self-worth, and small numbers only matter when you're considering interest rates. Listen, there are no rewards in Heaven for designer labels in size 8. There are rewards for appreciating the body you are currently in. Every size body can enjoy affordable clothes. Let your appreciation for things you don't have inspire you to be creative with the gifts already available in your life now.

4. Timidity

Opening up your closet door and seeing your prom dress and your wedding dress alongside the getting-back-into-the-dating-world dress you bought after the divorce five years ago is depressing! What are you holding onto? You've moved on. So should your clothes. Stop doubting yourself — holding back, hesitating. Your life is before you! You're stuck in the past when you should be enjoying the present. Your timidity could be keeping you from meeting the right people, getting hired for the right job, or finding the right partner. When life moves on, so must your wardrobe.

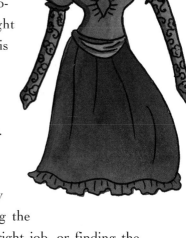

5. Comparison

Comparing your hips to Cindy Crawford's, your hair to Jennifer Aniston's, or your arms to the arms of your best friend is an awful habit. Comparing yourself to someone else is a poisonous cocktail from which you do not want to sip. You must resist the temptation to indulge in the act of comparing. Don't be seduced by airbrushed pictures of Hollywood stars that appear on glossy paper. It's all illusion! Everyone has cellulite. What you think your friend has in muscle tone, you make up for in tenaciousness (and your eyes are great too!).

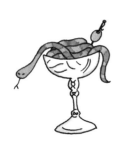

The fiery furnace of comparison will consume your self-esteem every time. It'll keep you from ever enjoying clothes on your own "perfect-as-is" body. You have your own set of gifts, talents, and assets that are unique to you and are begging to be appreciated and expressed. Stop comparing. Learn to focus on your assets and let them shine!

6. Settling

Compromising your desires can be a crushing blow to your spirit. You know how you go to the store to buy a white blouse and instead of buying the one you love, you settle for one that's okay, will do in a pinch, kinda works? "Settling" for something ends up feeling like undigested oatmeal sitting at the bottom of your stomach. Don't settle for an okay pant when a fantastic one is just another rack or store over from where you're standing.

7. Self-Denial

It's false humility to think that it's vain to focus on yourself and your clothing needs. Self-denial won't get you to Heaven. Expressing your true self will. Think about it. Is it "too showy" for a rose bush to produce beautiful roses? Is it self-indulgent for the sun to come up every day and glow so brightly for all to enjoy? Is it vain for you to look like your beautiful self? NO! The whole world benefits from your caring for yourself. Don't deny yourself the pleasure of looking and feeling your best.

Comparison, neglect, idolatry, timidity, delusion, settling, self-denial — **vow right now to call these fashion sins by their real names.** Recognize how they've kept you down and trampled your joy. Love yourself and walk away from the temptation to engage in them. It might not be easy. It takes practice, but you can triumph.

Here's something that can help — the Ten Fashion Commandments. By practicing them, you will find yourself on a clear path to self-love, self-acceptance, and happiness. When you accessorize according to these Fashion Commandment pearls, everything will look great on you! Put your sunglasses on because you're about to see

the fashion light!

the
ten fashion
commandments

1. Wear Only What You Love

It's out there. Find it. Wearing anything
less won't feel nearly as good.

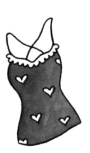

2. Make Clothes Personal

Dress yourself from the inside out. You don't have to dress like
your friends, your mother, or the models in fashion magazines.
Please yourself. Do you like silk, satin . . . or nubby textured
wool? Do you love primary colors . . . or prefer
pastels or neutrals? Do you love red cowboy
boots . . . backless pointy-toed mules . . . or
flowered flip-flops? It's your right to buy
lacy underwear, wear scarves that express
your fun sense of color, or dress in head-to-toe
black all day, every day, if that's what you like.

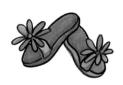

You don't have to be in what's "in" if what's "in" doesn't suit you.

3. Design and Develop a Wardrobe

That way you can have more time for fun. It takes time initially to identify what you love, to organize your closet, put outfits together that thrill you, and shop for the things you need, but once you do, you're free to be more involved in your life and less focused on how you look. It's because you've handled it. It's a lot like funding your retirement account. You do it and it's done. When your wardrobe covers your needs, you don't have to be worried about what to wear.

4. Concentrate on Your Assets

Suddenly your (perceived) liabilities will diminish. You have assets. Everyone does. No matter who you are or what you look like, you've been gifted with qualities that make you unique and beautiful. Invest your thoughts and actions in them. If you have a sexy, pouty mouth, dress it up in the perfect lipstick color. If you have broad, strong shoulders, show them off in halter tops. The world needs your particular variety of beauty. Don't hide your beauty under a barrel. Make it your passion to explore ways to celebrate it.

5. Dress the Body You Are Currently In

Don't put off dressing your body because you're waiting for it to change size. And don't wait for the time to be right either. You have the right body right now and the timing is perfect. Spend money on yourself now instead of waiting for the lottery to be won or the kids to be out of the house. You deserve to be happy right now just as you are in clothes that you love, that love you back.

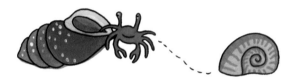

6. Focus on Fit, Not Size

Sometimes it takes the patience of Job to find the right fit, but have faith. Good fit is out there. Keep trying things on. If the garment doesn't fit, remember, it's the fault of the garment, not your body. Try on 30 pairs of jeans to find the fit and style you like best. Eleanor Roosevelt once said, "You must do the thing you think you cannot do." I know what she was talking about. She was talking about going to a dressing room with tops in three sizes and choosing the one that fits the best, not the one that has the size you like best. Do whatever it takes (getting a good tailor, shopping where a tailor is provided and alteration fees are free or nominal) to get good at recognizing good fit.

7. Don't Save Good Things for Good

Good is right now. It always has been and always will be. Why not wear your favorite blouse with your jeans when you go to the market? Why not put on that lipstick color you love so much as you head out to your kid's soccer game? Why not wear your best sweater to a movie? Looking good makes you feel good, no matter what.

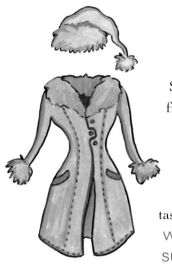

8. Keep Current

When life changes, change your clothes. Some of us leave a job that's formal and find a job that's casual. Some of us move to snow country, some of us move to Florida. All of us get older, and what was appropriate in our 20s usually doesn't cut it when we're 45. Our tastes and desires change over time. So, when life takes its turns, make sure your wardrobe turns with you. Remember to care for yourself and your wardrobe like you care for others — with patience, love, and devotion.

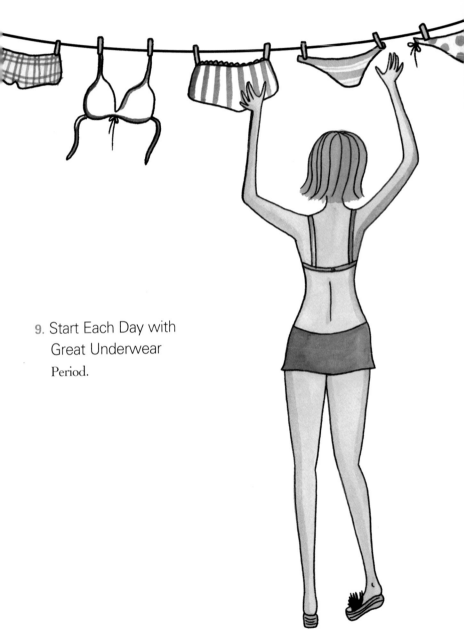

9. Start Each Day with
   Great Underwear

   Period.

10. End Each Day with Great Gratitude

You'll enjoy yourself, your life, and your wardrobe when you appreciate what you have. It's the key to happiness. Gratitude makes clothes hang better on you, makes you sleep better, and good sleep keeps you beautiful. You are blessed immeasurably, but measure at least three of those blessings a day — out loud, on paper, or whispered to your pillow before you go to sleep. It's the formula that works for getting true beauty rest.

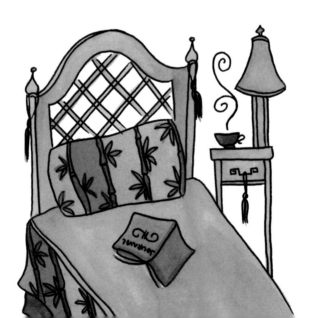

If you read these Ten Fashion Commandments regularly — the way people pray, meditate, and eat chocolate — they will ring gently in your ears, encouraging you to develop new, improved habits that will become as natural as breathing. When you're facing the jewelry counter, for instance, wondering which necklace to buy, you'll choose the one you love over the one that you would have "settled" for in the past. Reading the commandments often, as goals, will improve the chances that you'll be living the good life in the right clothes. So keep these handy,

refer to them often,

and your wardrobe will be transformed!

in the confessional with brenda

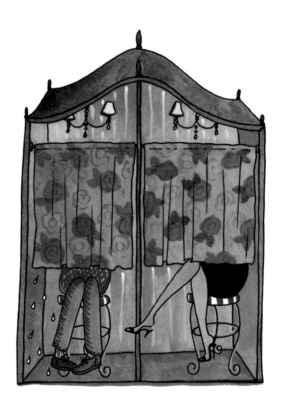

One benefit of listening to others' horror stories is getting tips about what NOT to do yourself. Like, when you show up for a meeting and it's snowing outside, it's best when you walk in the door to find a mirror to make sure your makeup isn't running down your chin. Wet black mascara tracks don't make a good impression. Or, you can learn which tailor to avoid because he lost another friend's pants, or what store to avoid because the salespeople talked about another friend while she was in the dressing room.

Some things are too painful to talk about, even to close friends, but in the privacy of a confessional booth, women feel free to spill the beans. Shhh ... Come on in. My confessional booth is decorated in peachy/pink-colored chintz drapes because that color looks good on every skin tone! Maybe by eavesdropping on other women's problems, yours will be lifted up into the heavens and disappear for good. Listen with a compassionate heart. Remember, this could be YOU in the confessional.

maria: Okay, so I went shopping and brought everything home, went to put my new things in the closet, and I bought everything that is already in there! I love black turtleneck sweaters and wooly pants, but I seem to have bought even more black turtlenecks and wooly pants. It's time to try something different, but now I'm too embarrassed to go back to the salesperson who helped me and return everything.

brenda: You're allowed to change your mind. It's one of the redemptions you have in life, especially if you shop in stores that pride themselves on their return policy — and return policies are definitely something to be aware of. Return policies are part of customer service, and if you aren't satisfied with your purchases you're supposed to take them back. If it's easier, bring a friend with you. If you feel compelled to offer an explanation, tell the salesperson what you just told me. I find the truth is always the best. If she's a good sales associate, she'll be interested in keeping you as a customer and being sure you're satisfied. If she's not, maybe you shouldn't be shopping with her.

maria: Can't I just make something up like my husband had a fit or my mother died and I need to pay for the funeral instead?

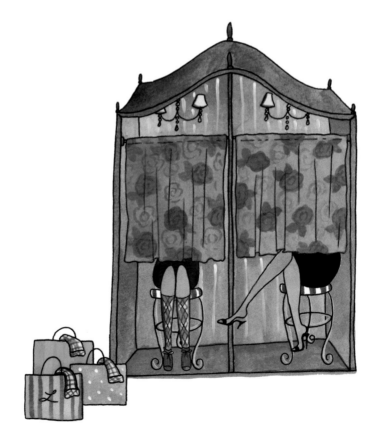

brenda: That might work once, but if you're the type who needs time to make decisions, you're going to have to keep coming up with lies, and that's complicated. Tell the sales associate that you really appreciate the policy of the store, but keep the focus on yourself. You're spending money on clothes to please yourself, not a salesperson. You're going to be wearing these things, not her. Stay the course.

catherine: Brenda, I'm a clothes hoarder. I shop and I shop and I shop. I've filled every closet in my house. I'm overtaking the bathtub for more storage. I don't want anyone to come over to my house and see this. I feel so ashamed. And yet, it still doesn't feel like it's enough. What's wrong with me?

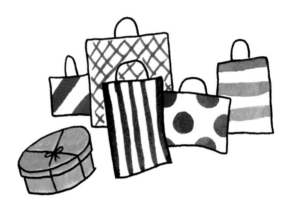

brenda: You could be overbuying to compensate for feeling "not enough" inside. And if that's the case, no number of clothes will fill that hole. Or you may be using shopping to avoid something big that you really want in your life but are side-stepping the need to find it — like the right livelihood, the right partner, or the right place to live. Whatever the bigger problem, shopping isn't going to fix it. Other people who have these problems have gotten help from therapists or groups that deal with shopping addictions. Find a professional therapist or get help from a 12-Step group like Debtors Anonymous. Their website is www.debtorsanonymous.org.

rhonda: Brenda, I have shopper's block. Shopping overwhelms me. I don't have a clue where to shop or what to look for. I don't even know what size I am or what I like. I don't belong in the clothes that live in my closet. They're out-of-date, but I don't know where to start! It seems like everyone knows how to do this but me.

brenda: You already know what's not working. Knowing what you dislike is very valuable information. Make a list of what you don't like. Everything. Now make a list of the current things you love. So, red cowboy boots are on that list? That's the place to start! If you're wild about those boots, then make them the focal piece and build outfits around them. Jeans and simple pants will show them off. Nice T-shirts and crisp blouses, a leather jacket plus a scarf that has some red in it (which will bring our eye up from the boots to your face) would be great. That's where you start. Start with what you love.

rhonda: But isn't that frivolous?

brenda: Is it frivolous to love? No! Here's a guiding light to help you remember this: Wear what you love, love what you wear. Always remember that guiding light, and you're on the road to happiness.

margie: I go to clean out my closet but I get hung up on all the things that people have given me. I can't say no to my friend who wants to give me all her hand-me-downs. We don't have the same coloring, don't share the same style, and don't even wear the same size! I hate to say no to her, but how can I be "me" when I open my closet and all I see are things that were hers!

brenda: If you can't say no to others, then at least make those clothes exit the same door they came in through. Out, out, all of them out! Go through every single thing in your closet and drawers and eliminate what doesn't fit you, attract you, enhance, or thrill you. Your rejects (and everyone else's) can reincarnate at the consignment store, a charity, or the curb. But ultimately, I suggest you stand up for yourself and tell the truth. Other people's rejects aren't your treasures just because you wish it were so. Kindly reject the offer of rejects. Tell you friend to take them to a charity instead. A charity, or the curb.

linda: Brenda, I can't go shopping with my best friend because I can never look as good in clothes as she does. She's beautiful in everything she tries on.

brenda: Ouch! That hurts. First of all, the only thing that's important when you're shopping is that you find clothes that you love, that love you back. If you're focused on that, you won't be focused on your best friend. There might be a buddy you enjoy shopping with more than your best friend, but if you could get past the deadly sin of comparing yourself to someone else, could your best friend be helpful to you? Remember this guiding light: Clothing is a tool for expressing your inner life. Turn your focus to your insides, to the qualities about yourself that you'd like to bring out. Maybe your best friend could help you identify that. After all, she's crazy about you. How about sensuality? Power? Warmth? Creativity?* What's your inner beauty that wants to be expressed right now? You have physical assets to highlight, absolutely, but you also have parts of your personality that are unique to you and those parts need expressing too. Think about this and get to work! It'll feel like play.

kathy: I buy everything on sale. I can't imagine paying full price for anything. My parents never did. I'd be breaking the family creed if I didn't wait for things to go on sale. My new friend, Margaret, never waits for sales. She has a budget but buys nice things she wears all the time, and she always looks great. Am I missing something here?

* See *Brenda's Wardrobe Companion,* the Style Glossary, for help in dressing inner qualities.

brenda: Be willing to release the family creed and deliver yourself from sale-shopping mentality. There is redeeming value in the cost-per-wear formula. If you buy a jacket for $300 and wear it 300 times, it cost you one dollar per wearing. If you buy a cheaper one for $50 and wear it once (because you didn't really LOVE it, but it was on sale), it cost you $50 per wear. I have a shopping mantra: You're worth full price! Remember that, and remember the cost-per-wear formula. You'll soon discover that you don't have to buy everything on sale to get great value.

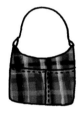

suzanne: I'm terrified of accessories. I go to tie a scarf and it comes out looking like a noose. Necklaces get tangled up in my jewelry box, and I want to dump the whole thing in the trash. I don't know if I'm supposed to wear a belt on my waist or on my hips. Can't I just forget about accessories?

brenda: Sometimes we must walk through the fire to enhance our clothes, and this is one of those times. Your clothes can only do so much for you, and then it's time to call in the accessories to add polish and personality to your outfit so you shine your unique light. Accessory terror is curable. First of all, people who work in accessory departments are usually very knowledgeable and passionate people. I predict there will be a shopping angel in a store of your liking who will happily simplify this part of dressing for you. Another thing you can do to be less accessory phobic is to get yourself to a fashion show. You don't have to go to Paris or Milan. Stores and charities often have fashion shows every season. Find one. Then pay attention to how the outfits are accessorized. Notice what attracts you. Jot down ideas. Maybe necklaces aren't your thing, but you love bracelets. Perhaps scarves don't resonate for you, but distinctive handbags do. Find things you love and play. Remember this pearl of wisdom: Accessorize to individualize. It's also possible that your fear of accessories is really avoidance of finishing an outfit. Often people get into ruts, buy the clothes that are easy to buy, but consequently never finish an outfit. Trust me, this will be good for you. Completing an outfit is as satisfying as completing a cross-word puzzle, a gourmet meal, or a work or art. Don't flake out on yourself. You deserve to look great from head to toe.

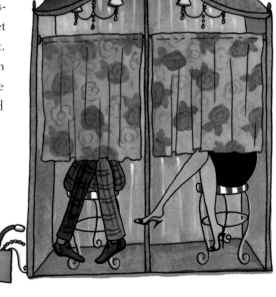

mary: Okay, so I was never a good shopper to begin with, but now I don't even *want* to go near the stores since I lost my favorite thing, my waistline.

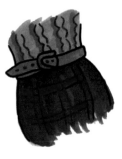

 brenda: Wait, let me guess. You'll only consider shopping again when you lose ten pounds, right?

mary: Right; at least then it would be fun again.

 brenda: Mary, my friend, remember the Fifth Commandment and shop for the body you are currently in. You and I don't know if that waistline will ever return, and you're worshipping it as though it's a god or something. Worship something else, like the idea of looking good right now, just as you are. Walking around lusting after something you once had only makes life hell. Get out there and celebrate that beautiful hair and those long legs! Enjoy focusing on your assets. Pick three things you want to highlight, and then dress so those three things show up. A boatneck sweater will highlight a nice shoulder line. A slim pant and slender boots with heels will make those legs look so long. A necklace that incorporates your eye color will have everyone complimenting you all day long on your gorgeous eyes. And in the meantime, while your waistline is hanging back from the spotlight, be sure to dress in clothes that bathe that waistline in comfort. Adopt this mantra: Fit first. It doesn't matter what size you have on, focus on the fit.

patty: I feel so dumpy! I look at my size 8 pants and I remember how sexy I felt in them. I'll probably never fit in pants like that again and I feel so bad!

brenda: It's time to redefine sexy. Sexy is a state of mind that has nothing to do with pants size. In fact, I'd guess that wearing a size bigger, as long as it's a flattering cut, will make you still feel that same way. Just having clothes that fit make you feel so much sexier than clothes that bind. There are so many ways to look fetching. Focus on a new way. Show some skin. Somewhere. Maybe a deep v-neck to show off your pretty cleavage. Or maybe you have a long neck that's very sexy. Wear long dangly earrings. Wear red lipstick or add some false eyelashes that look natural and enhance your own. Pull your hair up with hair ornaments and let a few strands drift down. Polish your nails and your toes. Wear open-toed shoes. Wear shiny fabrics. There are at least half a dozen things you can do at any given time that will say, "Sexy!" Every woman on earth — no matter her size — can express her sensual nature. Try thinking sexy to be sexy. Put a bounce in your step. Pull your shoulders back. Be proud. You're a woman and that's gorgeous!

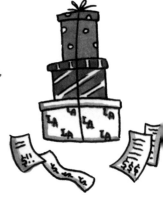

deborah: I really feel weird saying this, but I feel bad for loving clothes so much. I feel ashamed that it's so important to me to have nice things. Sometimes I think I should give up my lust for clothes and join a convent.

brenda: Oh boy, you've got the guilties and they aren't in your colors! Enjoying nice things is just one aspect of you. It's not the "all" of you. Can you accept that the same way you accept that you're good at math and enjoy solving problems or that you have a way with dogs and can get them to behave? Your love of clothes just "is." Don't judge it, and don't reject it either. It'll just keep coming up like burps after a spicy meal. Let your love of nice things live comfortably in you. It's okay.

deborah: Well, is there a way to have nice-looking things without spending a fortune? That way, I can give to my favorite charities too.

brenda: Absolutely. It helps to understand how fashion works. Fashion starts on runways in Milan, Paris, London, and New York. The clothes are expensive and exaggerated, and you and I will never buy or wear those clothes. But, the trickle-down theory works with fashion

— only it's turned into a rushing-waterfall theory. The minute those fashions leave the runways, they are being copied by lower-end manufacturers and will appear in your major department stores in a few weeks, not exactly the same designs, but close . . . more wearable, in less expensive fabrics. But if something is trendy, it doesn't need to be in a forever fabric because you're not going to wear it forever. It's going to be your one-season wonder. Here's a good trick: At the beginning of a fashion season, go to the most expensive departments of a store and check out the clothes. Even try things on. It's okay if the pant is $3000. You're just looking at the silhouette and the details. Once your mind is imprinted with what the current looks are from the top

designers, you can go to the lower-end departments and stores and find the look. Nearly all fashion magazines now devote a few pages to showing you the real and the look-alikes for less. Pick up some magazines and 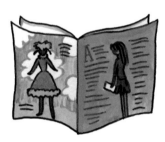 steal their ideas.

They want you to!

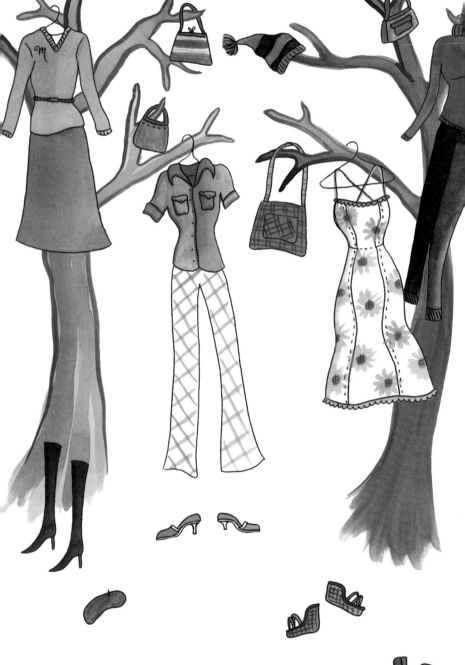

to everything there is a
fashion season

It is said that the world was created in seven days —
well, six actually. The seventh day was a day of rest.
Resting is good. You'll have great rest and loads of
satisfaction when you don't have to worry about
clothes. But in order to do that, you have to devote
some time and attention to your wardrobe now before
you're in dire need of something and run the risk of
"terror shopping." That's when you run out at the
last minute and come home with who-knows-what
desperate thing you wear once and then never look at
again. There are steps to take to keep desperation out
of your life. Take them one season at a time.

Start at the beginning of the calendar year. Here's
what you need to do.

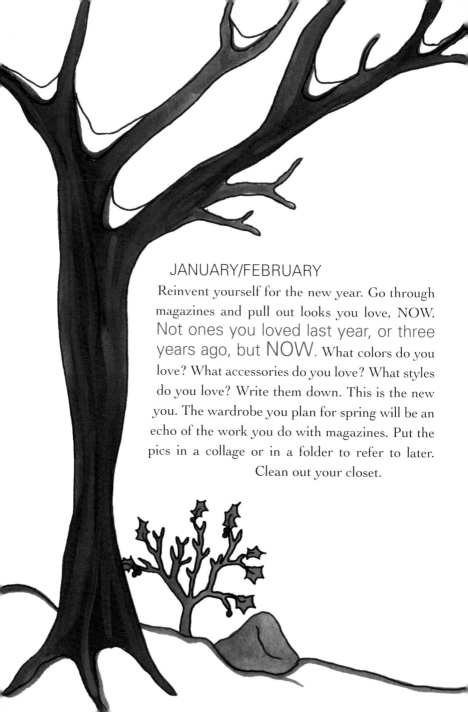

JANUARY/FEBRUARY

Reinvent yourself for the new year. Go through magazines and pull out looks you love, NOW. Not ones you loved last year, or three years ago, but NOW. What colors do you love? What accessories do you love? What styles do you love? Write them down. This is the new you. The wardrobe you plan for spring will be an echo of the work you do with magazines. Put the pics in a collage or in a folder to refer to later.

Clean out your closet.

STEP 1:

Get out everything that doesn't fit or just isn't right for you any longer. You know what they are! Confess! Make room for the things you love to wear so you can see them and choose them. Try on all the clothes in your closet that you plan to wear this upcoming season — spring/summer. Divide them into "what stays" and "what goes."

STEP 2:

Take an inventory. What do you need to fill into your wardrobe? Start making a master shopping list of what you need and want to add to your wardrobe.

STEP 3:

Look ahead four months and see what's coming up in your life. Do you have weddings to go to? Graduations? Out-of-town business conventions? Write down all the things you need clothes for. Go to your closet and see if you have the right clothes for special occasions. If not, add them to your master shopping list.

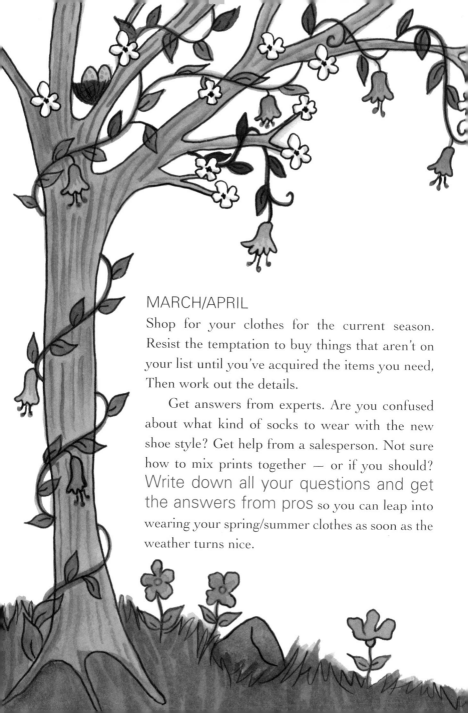

MARCH/APRIL

Shop for your clothes for the current season. Resist the temptation to buy things that aren't on your list until you've acquired the items you need, Then work out the details.

Get answers from experts. Are you confused about what kind of socks to wear with the new shoe style? Get help from a salesperson. Not sure how to mix prints together — or if you should? Write down all your questions and get the answers from pros so you can leap into wearing your spring/summer clothes as soon as the weather turns nice.

MAY/JUNE
"Finish" everything.

STEP 1:

Go get your makeup done at a makeup counter in a department store, or make an appointment with an in-home service such as Mary Kay Cosmetics. Makeup colors have seasons, just like clothes. So every spring and fall you can make color adjustments that will also make your whole wardrobe feel fresh and new, even if you aren't shopping for any new clothes that season. A new lipstick color works miracles to freshen up a wardrobe that's not seeing many changes in a given season.

STEP 2:

Review your hairstyle and color. Learn about hair products designed to remedy your specific problems and help you manage a great look. Learn something new, and then practice doing that new thing. Let your hair go curly or learn how to use a blow dryer. It'll keep you feeling young and refreshed. And don't hide your beauty behind a hairstyle that is too dated for you.

STEP 3:

Accessorize, accessorize, accessorize. Now that you've shopped for your clothes, be sure you have the right shoes, handbags, hair ornaments, jewelry, and hats to personalize your look.

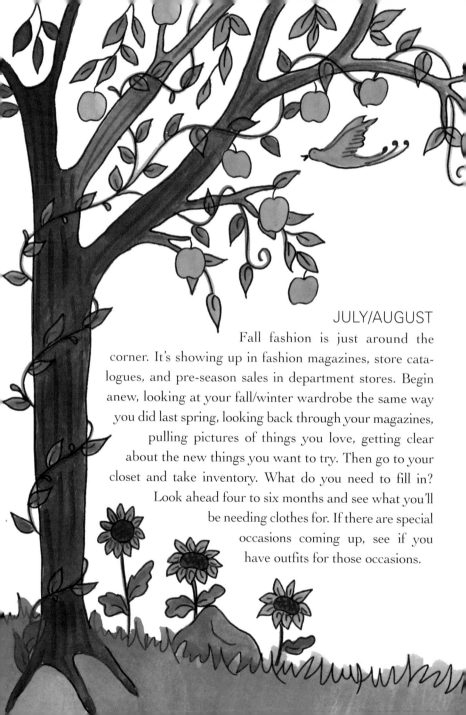

JULY/AUGUST

Fall fashion is just around the corner. It's showing up in fashion magazines, store catalogues, and pre-season sales in department stores. Begin anew, looking at your fall/winter wardrobe the same way you did last spring, looking back through your magazines, pulling pictures of things you love, getting clear about the new things you want to try. Then go to your closet and take inventory. What do you need to fill in? Look ahead four to six months and see what you'll be needing clothes for. If there are special occasions coming up, see if you have outfits for those occasions.

SEPTEMBER/OCTOBER

Shop for your fall/winter clothes. If you are shopping for holiday clothes, expect to shop for those in late October. Have your makeup reviewed with "fall" in mind. Expect to change your makeup colors to work with the season.

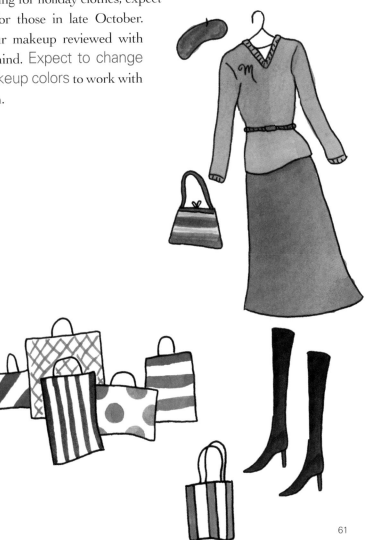

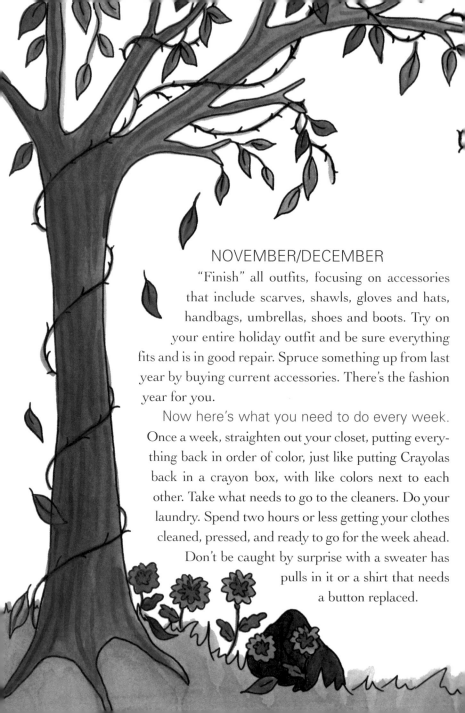

NOVEMBER/DECEMBER

"Finish" all outfits, focusing on accessories that include scarves, shawls, gloves and hats, handbags, umbrellas, shoes and boots. Try on your entire holiday outfit and be sure everything fits and is in good repair. Spruce something up from last year by buying current accessories. There's the fashion year for you.

Now here's what you need to do every week. Once a week, straighten out your closet, putting everything back in order of color, just like putting Crayolas back in a crayon box, with like colors next to each other. Take what needs to go to the cleaners. Do your laundry. Spend two hours or less getting your clothes cleaned, pressed, and ready to go for the week ahead.

Don't be caught by surprise with a sweater has pulls in it or a shirt that needs a button replaced.

And here's what you do **every day**:

STEP 1:

Put yourself first every morning.
Don't do everything else first then
rush yourself into the shower.
Take time to put on your makeup,
style your hair and choose your
clothes with joy.

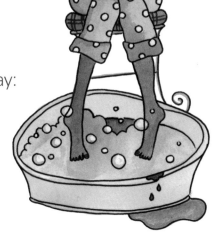

STEP 2:

Look at yourself in a full-length mirror before you walk out the
door. Are all the hems where they're supposed to be? Are you
dressed appropriately for the activities of the day? Don't forget
to check out your backside.

STEP 3:

Leave the house wearing what you love. And if it's the same outfit every day, fine. That's very European, and those Europeans
know fashion! Or if at first you don't love everything you're
wearing, start with one thing you're just mad for and build from
there.

STEP 4:

Always wear lipstick!

STEP 5:

At the end of the day, spend a minute with your gratitude list.
Count your blessings into your pillow. You are truly blessed!

miracle
makeovers

You may never be the winner of a makeover for a national TV show, but that doesn't mean you can't experience some miracle makeovers of your own right now.

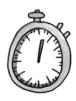

1. One-Second Makeover
Add a smile to your outfit. It doesn't cost a thing. And it's completely transforming for you and all the lucky people who receive it.

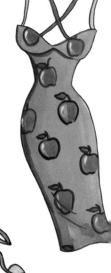

2. Ten-Second Makeover
Stand up straight, drop your shoulders, open your heart. This not only changes your look, it changes how you look at things.

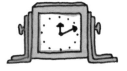

3. Ten-Minute Makeover to Look Ten Pounds Thinner

Fill in your eyebrows. Lift your bra straps and loosen your belt. Wear a size bigger to look a size smaller. Add a pretty lipstick color and the extra bounce in your step will be automatic.

4. One-Hour Accessory Makeover

Pick a favorite trend and find it in a shoe, scarf, handbag, or piece of jewelry. Add it to last year's outfit to look completely current. The crystal necklace, the paisley scarf, the orange and purple plaid handbag is the fashion "pow" that creates this moment's big "wow." It doesn't matter what age you are; sprinkling your wardrobe with trends is dipping into the fountain of youth. So refreshing!

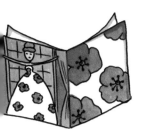

5. Ten-Hour Makeover to be Reborn

Grab a stack of magazines. Pull out pictures of things you love. Identify what you love about them. Make a list of those things. Drive to the nearest store. Engage a friendly salesperson or bring a shopping buddy to help you shop for what you love. Put together the look from head to toe in one outfit. Call a friend, go to a club, and watch the heads turn.

heaven
on earth

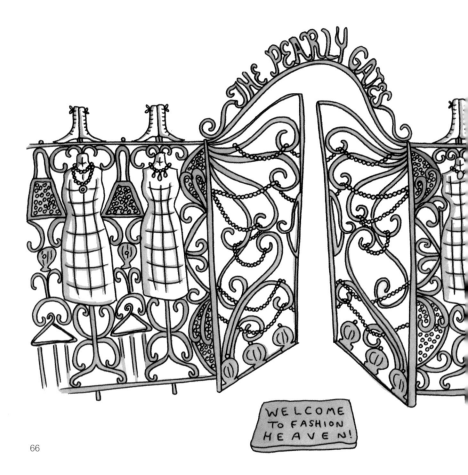

When you're no longer tempted by the Seven Deadly Fashion Sins — and you train yourself to follow the Ten Fashion Commandments, you'll get your fashion wings. You'll be experiencing fashion epiphanies all over town. You'll notice when you make time to think about your clothes ahead of time, you can participate more happily in your life. With your clothes taken care of you can get on with important matters. That's when you've found fashion heaven right here on earth.

Need some inspiration while you're making progress? Read ahead to these letters from women who reside in Paradise. They'll show you the stair steps to fashion heaven.

Dear Brenda,

I've become a good customer of an alterations person who helps me fine-tune the fit of my clothes so they softly grace and flatter me. One of my hips is higher than the other, and she makes just the right adjustments every time. One shoulder is higher, too, and she'll knows to adjust one sleeve length but not the other. It's great to understand my body better and how to make clothes fit.

Signed,
Finally Fitting In

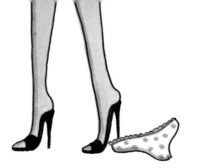

Step 2. Let Go

Dear Brenda,

Since I got rid of my expired clothes, getting dressed every morning is a breeze. My clothes are organized by color, which makes it so easy to see what's in there. Because there's nothing in there that I don't love, there's actually space between the hangers. Now, if my husband wants more time with me in the morning, I know that I can have fun with him and still be dressed in five minutes. Having only clothes in my closet that fit my life now has saved all kinds of time and energy.

Signed,
Satisfied Over
and Over

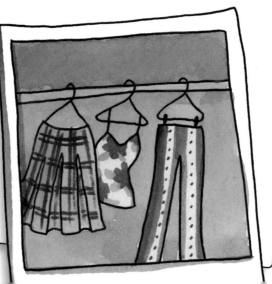

Step 3. Try Something New

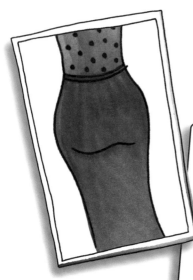

Dear Brenda,

I never thought I'd be fifty and wearing thong underwear, but my daughter said, "Mom, just try them for two weeks and you'll never go back to the granny briefs." She was right! And now I never worry about panty lines. I love how I look from the back. Wow, it's never too late to learn something new about myself in clothes.

Signed,
Younger at 50 Than at 30

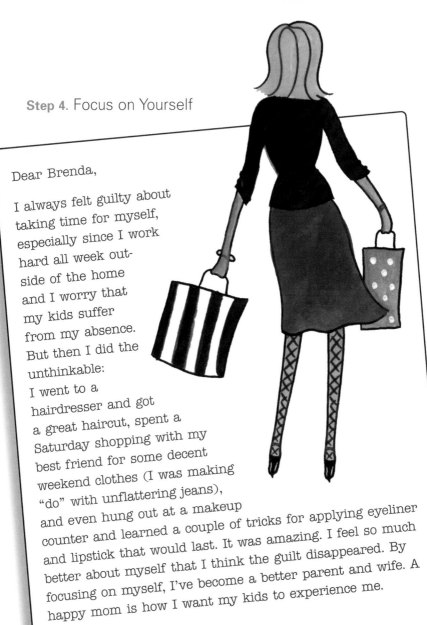

Dear Brenda,

I always felt guilty about taking time for myself, especially since I work hard all week outside of the home and I worry that my kids suffer from my absence. But then I did the unthinkable: I went to a hairdresser and got a great haircut, spent a Saturday shopping with my best friend for some decent weekend clothes (I was making "do" with unflattering jeans), and even hung out at a makeup counter and learned a couple of tricks for applying eyeliner and lipstick that would last. It was amazing. I feel so much better about myself that I think the guilt disappeared. By focusing on myself, I've become a better parent and wife. A happy mom is how I want my kids to experience me.

Signed, A Pretty Parent

Dear Brenda,

I used to be so confused. I would dress to please my mother-in-law, my husband, or my own mom, but I never felt right in my clothes. Then I said, "Enough already! I want to figure out what I like." Now when I go shopping, I only buy what makes me see more of myself than I've seen before and not more of the person my mother wished I was. I'm so much happier!

Signed,
Free To Be Me

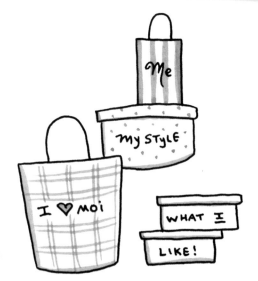

Step 6. Get a Healthy Perspective

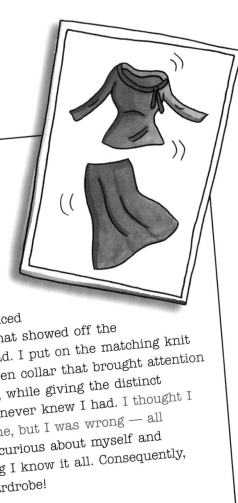

Dear Brenda,

I was convinced that I had no waist and short legs. My solution was to hide my shape, wear boxy jackets and pleated pants. Then I was shopping with my shopping buddy who convinced me to put on a knit skirt that showed off the shapely calves I forgot I had. I put on the matching knit top with sleeves and an open collar that brought attention to the top half of my body, while giving the distinct appearance of the waist I never knew I had. I thought I knew what was best for me, but I was wrong — all wrong. I've decided to be curious about myself and clothes instead of thinking I know it all. Consequently, I'm delighted with my wardrobe!

Signed,
Thinking Curvy Thoughts

Dear Brenda,

Ever since I gained some weight, I'm getting all this attention for how I look. It's the weirdest thing! I used to think I'd have to be a perfect size in order to look good. But I'm happy with my shape now that I've accepted my curves. I'm just wearing what I love, and it's sending out a positive message.

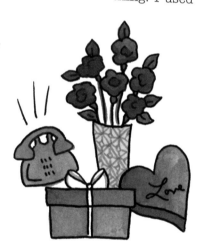

Signed,
Looking "Wow"
at Any Size or Age

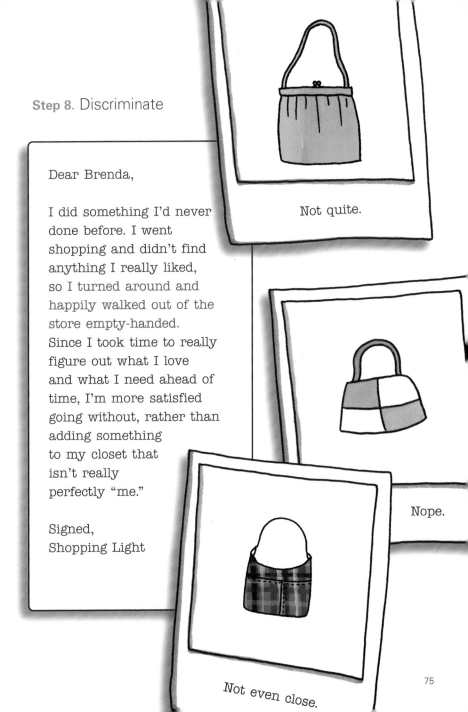

Step 8. Discriminate

Not quite.

Dear Brenda,

I did something I'd never done before. I went shopping and didn't find anything I really liked, so I turned around and happily walked out of the store empty-handed. Since I took time to really figure out what I love and what I need ahead of time, I'm more satisfied going without, rather than adding something to my closet that isn't really perfectly "me."

Signed,
Shopping Light

Nope.

Not even close.

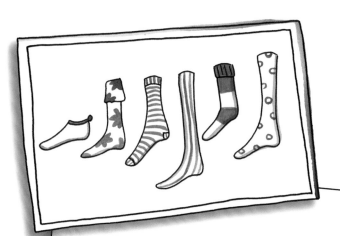

Dear Brenda,

I went through my wardrobe this fall and filled in all the gaps. As a result, I spent the whole season enjoying all of my clothes. In the past, I'd never have had the right socks to wear with my shoes until it was time to bring out my sandals for summer. I actually made my appearance a priority. I made it a project with a checklist and got it done. By handling it early, I'm enjoying great outfits all season long.

Signed,
Got It Handled

Dear Brenda,

I used to be so jealous of my friend Nancy who looks good in everything. But then one day I decided that maybe I could learn something from her. So I studied her habits. She doesn't really have many clothes, they are just the "right" clothes for her. She always goes out the door with makeup on. Her hairstyle is simple, but always well-groomed. Her shoes are always in great shape. So is her handbag. When I dissected what made her look great, I saw that I could imitate her habits with results that made me happy. Now I don't put myself down anymore. I'm taking much better care of myself. And I'm getting all sorts of compliments. Style can be learned! Just copy the work of the masters.

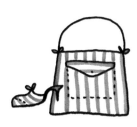

Signed,
Green Eyes for Beauty

FINAL WORDS

People who have languished in fashion hell for years, deprived of self-love and self-acceptance, will experience nothing short of delight when they open the doors to receive their beauty and let the light shine in. When you dress from the inside out, working with your assets, making your body right, and wearing what you love, you'll have joy beyond measure. You'll open your closet and everything in there will be saying, "Wear me! Wear me today!" Getting dressed will be one of your most satisfying experiences each day.

If you find yourself occasionally lost, and you fear you're in Purgatory, go back. Study the Commandments again, and find a deeper message that's there for you, something you missed the first time around. Ask yourself where you've committed a fashion sin, and if you got snagged there, simply confess. Be kind to yourself. Just by recognizing old habits you are free to make better choices.

If life provides a shakeup — like a move, a job change, a divorce, or a death in the family — and you're questioning your identity, go back to the beginning of the Fashion Season and do the work of figuring out who you are and what you love now. It's always so lovely to cultivate your uniqueness. Celebrate you!

Keep evolving. Every year is a new year. Every season is a new season. There are infinite ways to discover yourself. Experience the powerful way that clothes can remind you of who you are, who you are becoming, and who you have become every day. Nurture your nature with clothes that fit and flatter, and spotlight the splendor of your being.

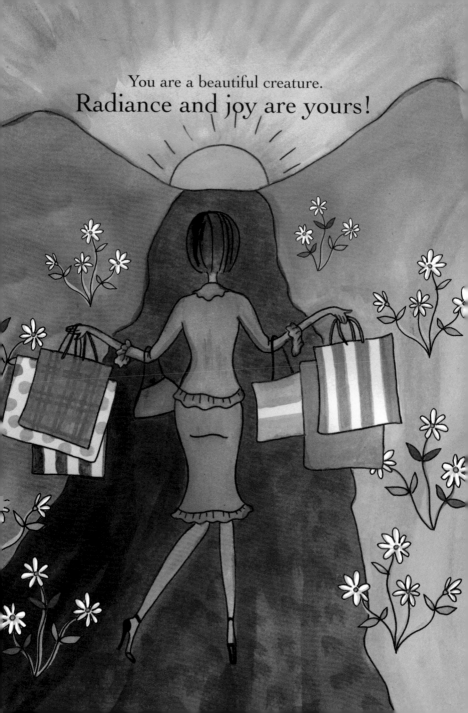

You are a beautiful creature.
Radiance and joy are yours!